The 21-Day Low Sodium Diet Plan for Women Over 50

A Beginner's Guide to Managing Heart Health and Energy With Simple Recipes and a Meal Plan

mf

copyright © 2025 Mary Golanna

All rights reserved No part of this book may be reproduced, or stored in a retrieval system, or transmitted in any form or by any means, electronic, mechanical, photocopying, recording, or otherwise, without express written permission of the publisher.

Disclaimer

By reading this disclaimer, you are accepting the terms of the disclaimer in full. If you disagree with this disclaimer, please do not read the guide.

All of the content within this guide is provided for informational and educational purposes only, and should not be accepted as independent medical or other professional advice. The author is not a doctor, physician, nurse, mental health provider, or registered nutritionist/dietician. Therefore, using and reading this guide does not establish any form of a physician-patient relationship.

Always consult with a physician or another qualified health provider with any issues or questions you might have regarding any sort of medical condition. Do not ever disregard any qualified professional medical advice or delay seeking that advice because of anything you have read in this guide. The information in this guide is not intended to be any sort of medical advice and should not be used in lieu of any medical advice by a licensed and qualified medical professional.

The information in this guide has been compiled from a variety of known sources. However, the author cannot attest to or guarantee the accuracy of each source and thus should not be held liable for any errors or omissions.

You acknowledge that the publisher of this guide will not be held liable for any loss or damage of any kind incurred as a result of this guide or the reliance on any information provided within this guide. You acknowledge and agree that you assume all risk and responsibility for any action you undertake in response to the information in this guide.

Using this guide does not guarantee any particular result (e.g., weight loss or a cure). By reading this guide, you acknowledge that there are no guarantees to any specific outcome or results you can expect.

All product names, diet plans, or names used in this guide are for identification purposes only and are the property of their respective owners. The use of these names does not imply endorsement. All other trademarks cited herein are the property of their respective owners.

Where applicable, this guide is not intended to be a substitute for the original work of this diet plan and is, at most, a supplement to the original work for this diet plan and never a direct substitute. This guide is a personal expression of the facts of that diet plan.

Where applicable, persons shown in the cover images are stock photography models and the publisher has obtained the rights to use the images through license agreements with third-party stock image companies.

Table of Contents

Introduction	8
Understanding the Root Cause	10
Why Women Over 50 Are More Sensitive to Salt	10
The Link Between Sodium, Hormones, and Energy	12
What to Expect in the Next 21 Days	14
Why Salt Matters More After 50	17
Blood Pressure, Menopause & Sodium Retention	18
Hidden Salt Triggers for Fatigue	19
Where Salt Hides and How to Outsmart It	22
Where Sodium Hides	22
How to Outsmart Hidden Sodium	23
Common High-Sodium Foods at Home and Restaurants	24
At Home	24
How to Read Nutrition Labels After 50 (Even Without Glasses!)	26
What Happens When You Lower Sodium	29
Heart Health Benefits	30
Better Sleep, Less Bloating	32
Mood and Energy Boosts	33
The 21-Day Action Plan for Lowering Sodium	36
Prep Week: Set Yourself Up for Success	36
Week 1: Awareness & Reset	38
Low-Sodium Lentil Soup	44
Baked Salmon with Lemon and Dill	45
Week 2: Balance & Boost	47
Turkey and Avocado Wrap	54
Grilled Chicken Stir-Fry	55
Week 3: Lasting Habits	57
Garlic-Roasted Cod	64

Veggie-Packed Turkey Chili	65
Low-Sodium Recipe Toolkit	**68**
Comfort Foods Made Heart-Healthy	69
Low-Sodium Shepherd's Pie	69
Low-Sodium Vegetable Lasagna	71
Low-Sodium Sloppy Joes	72
Low-Sodium Chicken Alfredo	73
Heart-Healthy Mashed Potato Bowl	74
Quick Lunches for Energy	75
Zesty Quinoa Salad	75
Turkey and Avocado Wrap	76
Low-Sodium Tuna Salad	77
Caprese Salad with a Twist	78
Egg Salad Wrap	79
Batch Dinners for the Week	80
Stuffed Bell Peppers	80
Vegetable Stir-Fry	81
Slow Cooker Lentil Soup	82
Greek-Style Chicken Bowls	83
Turkey Meatballs in Tomato Sauce	84
Flavorful Dressings & Seasonings	85
Orange-Tahini Dressing	85
Garlic Herb Vinaigrette	86
Coconut Lime Dressing	87
Smoky Paprika Rub	88
Lemon-Dill Marinade	89
Guilt-Free Snacks	90
Carrot Sticks and Hummus	90
Nut-Free Energy Bites	91
Baked Sweet Potato Chips	92
Frozen Banana Coins	93

Apple Nachos	94
Maintaining a Low-Sodium, Heart-Healthy Lifestyle	**95**
How to Keep It Up After 21 Days	95
When You Don't Feel Like Cooking	96
Handling Parties, Travel & Family Pressure	97
Real-Life Maintenance Plan	98
Conclusion	**100**
FAQs	**103**
References and Helpful Links	**106**

Introduction

When you pass the milestone of 50, your body begins to go through profound changes. Hormonal shifts, like menopause, can affect how you process sodium, leaving you more prone to high blood pressure, fatigue, and bloating. On the flip side, staying in control of your sodium intake can help protect your heart, give you more energy, and make you feel vibrant again.

If you've felt overwhelmed by salt and aren't sure where to start, you're not alone. For women over 50, managing sodium can feel like a puzzle. This guide is here to help you solve it. With clear explanations, actionable tips, and recipes bursting with flavor (not salt), you'll have the tools to take charge.

In this guide, we will talk about the following:

- Understanding the Root Cause. We'll explore why salt becomes a bigger issue after 50 and how reducing it affects your health and energy.
- A 21-Day Action Plan to help you ease into a low-sodium lifestyle with meal plans, prep ideas, and small victories to keep you motivated.

- Recipes and Long-Term Support that help you sustain this way of eating, even when life throws challenges your way.

This guide walks you through everything you need—from understanding why salt impacts you more now than it did at 30, to a complete 21-day plan, and long-term strategies. You'll learn how to outsmart hidden sodium, cook delicious low-sodium meals, and boost both your energy and mood.

Keep reading to learn more about how to tackle the salt issue in your diet and improve your overall health. By the end, you'll have all the confidence you need to live well without sacrificing taste or convenience.

Understanding the Root Cause

Understanding the root cause is the first step in solving any problem effectively. By identifying the underlying issue, rather than just addressing symptoms, we can develop long-term solutions. In this chapter, we'll explore the importance of digging deeper and uncovering the true source of challenges.

Why Women Over 50 Are More Sensitive to Salt

If you're over 50, you might've noticed your body reacts differently to salty foods than it used to. Maybe your rings feel tighter, or you wake up with puffiness around your eyes. These changes aren't random and often come down to how your body processes salt as you age. Knowing what's happening can help you make small, simple changes to feel better and stay healthier.

1. **Hormones and Salt Retention**

    Before menopause, your body has an easier time handling salt thanks to a hormone called estrogen. This hormone helps your kidneys get rid of extra salt and keeps your body's fluids balanced. But after menopause, estrogen levels drop, making it harder for your body to process salt. This means you're more likely to hold on to sodium, which can cause bloating, puffiness, and even raised blood pressure.

This change in how your body deals with salt also affects your energy. Too much sodium can leave you feeling sluggish and drained, especially during the midday slump. It makes those low-energy moments feel even heavier.

2. How Too Much Salt Affects Your Heart

Over time, your blood vessels naturally become less flexible, which means they don't manage extra fluid as well as they used to. When you eat a lot of salt, your body holds onto water to balance it out, increasing the amount of fluid in your bloodstream. This puts extra pressure on your heart and blood vessels, which can raise your blood pressure. For women over 50, who are already at higher risk for heart problems after menopause, cutting back on sodium is a simple but powerful way to protect your health.

3. Signs That Too Much Salt Might Be a Problem

Your body often gives clear signals when it's holding onto too much sodium. Common signs include:

Swollen fingers or hands: Your rings might feel tight after eating something salty.

- ***Puffy face in the morning***: Salty meals the night before can leave you with noticeable puffiness around your eyes.
- ***Swollen feet or ankles***: After sitting for a long time, you might notice your socks leave deep marks around your legs.

Understanding how your body processes salt after 50 can help you make healthier choices and reduce uncomfortable symptoms like bloating and puffiness. By cutting back on sodium, you can support your heart health and feel more energized every day.

The Link Between Sodium, Hormones, and Energy

After menopause, your body undergoes several changes, including how it handles sodium and the impact this has on your energy levels. These changes are largely tied to the drop in estrogen, a hormone that plays a major role in keeping your body in balance.

Before menopause, estrogen helps your kidneys manage sodium efficiently. It works like a supportive partner, ensuring your body removes any extra salt and keeps your fluid levels stable. But as estrogen levels decrease, so does your body's ability to process sodium effectively. This often results in sodium staying in your system longer, leading to fluid retention and feelings of puffiness or bloating.

This retained sodium puts more strain on your system. By holding onto extra water, your blood volume increases, which can push your blood pressure higher. These adjustments, while subtle, can leave you feeling heavier and more fatigued. Your body has to work harder simply to maintain its equilibrium, which saps energy that could otherwise be used to get through your day.

On top of that, the hormonal shifts during menopause also create broader effects on how you feel. It's common to experience dips in energy or waves of sluggishness during this time. When sodium is added to the equation, it can amplify those lows and make recovery between energy dips even slower.

Understanding this connection between sodium, hormones, and energy is a key step in tuning into how your body is changing after menopause. By recognizing the role sodium plays, you can start to notice patterns in how certain foods or habits make you feel, empowering you to adjust and support steady, balanced energy levels.

What to Expect in the Next 21 Days

Making changes to your diet can feel intimidating, but sticking with a low-sodium plan for just three weeks can transform the way you feel. Here's an overview of how your body adapts during this time and the benefits to look forward to.

Week 1: Adjusting to Change

The first week is all about helping your body adapt. If you're used to the intense flavor of salty foods, meals might taste a little bland at first. This adjustment period happens because your taste buds are highly sensitive to salt after years of exposure. The good news? Your palate is adaptable and will recalibrate after a few days.

Here's what you might notice:

- *Less Bloating*: Cutting back on sodium reduces water retention, meaning you'll likely feel "lighter" within days.
- *More Hydration*: By drinking plenty of water and reducing salt, you'll experience a refreshing, hydrated feeling that keeps you energized.

Actionable Tip:

Focus on flavor rather than salt. Roast vegetables with olive oil and fresh thyme or toss salads with vinaigrettes made from lemon juice and mustard. These tweaks can make all the difference.

Week 2: Building Momentum

By the second week, your body is responding positively to less sodium. You're likely sleeping better and experiencing more consistent energy throughout the day. Many women also report a clearer mind and a brighter mood as their body stabilizes.

Here's where the magic starts:

- *Blood Pressure Benefits*: Early signs of improvement in blood pressure may show up, especially if you've also increased your potassium intake.
- *Better Taste Sensitivity*: Foods you once thought were bland may start to taste richer and more enjoyable.

Actionable Tip:

This is a great time to explore herbs and spices. Try using smoked paprika on roasted chicken or turmeric in rice to create bold, interesting flavors.

Week 3 and Beyond: A Lifestyle Shift

Week three is when everything starts to feel easier and more natural. Meals without added salt no longer feel like a sacrifice, and you might find yourself enjoying the vibrant, natural flavors of whole foods even more.

Long-term benefits become clearer as well:

- *Improved Heart Health*: Lowering sodium reduces strain on your heart and decreases your risk of hypertension.
- *Sustained Energy*: With less bloating and better sleep patterns, energy levels remain steady throughout the day.
- *Confidence in Choices*: By now, you'll feel more confident about reading labels, choosing low-sodium options, and creating satisfying meals at home.

Practical Tip:

Keep a list of your go-to low-sodium recipes and snacks. Familiarity is key to creating habits that stick. Keep ingredients like avocados, unsalted nuts, and fresh herbs on hand to make delicious meals or snacks quickly.

The beauty of this 21-day reset isn't just about what changes today; it's about setting the foundation for a heart-healthy, energized future. The empowerment that comes with taking control of your health and energy levels is invaluable. Even if you stumble along the way, every step forward is a win. With a little patience, creativity, and a focus on the flavors you love, this can be a sustainable lifestyle that helps you thrive well beyond 50.

Why Salt Matters More After 50

After the age of 50, your body undergoes many changes that can affect your heart and overall cardiovascular health. Your blood vessels naturally become less elastic, which means they don't expand and contract as effectively as they once did. At the same time, your heart may not work as efficiently at pumping blood. These changes are a natural part of aging, but they can be exacerbated by certain lifestyle factors, including a high-sodium diet.

Sodium plays a direct role in this equation because high levels can lead to increased fluid retention. When your body retains more water, it increases the volume of blood flowing through your vessels. This additional volume means your heart has to pump harder and your blood vessels are under more strain, which can elevate blood pressure. Over time, high blood pressure (or hypertension) damages the blood vessels and raises the risk of heart disease, stroke, and kidney problems.

By limiting your sodium intake, you're reducing the workload on your heart and vascular system. This simple but impactful change helps to regulate blood pressure and decrease inflammation in the body.

Blood Pressure, Menopause & Sodium Retention

After menopause, the body experiences a natural decline in estrogen levels, and this hormonal change directly impacts how your body retains sodium. Pre-menopause, estrogen helps regulate salt and water balance in the body, keeping sodium retention in check. But as estrogen levels drop, sodium retention becomes more pronounced. This means more water is held in the body, further contributing to high blood pressure.

This shift in sodium retention is one of the factors that make post-menopausal women more prone to hypertension. While high blood pressure isn't always accompanied by symptoms, its long-term effects can be serious, leading to increased risks of heart disease and strokes if left unchecked.

Steps to Address Sodium Retention

1. ***Stay Well-Hydrated***: It may seem counterintuitive, but drinking plenty of water can help combat sodium retention. When you're dehydrated, your body holds onto sodium even more to maintain its fluid balance. Aim for about 8–10 glasses of water a day, adjusting for your activity level and environment.

2. ***Reduce Processed and Packaged Foods***: Packaged snacks, frozen dinners, and pre-made sauces often contain large amounts of hidden sodium. A single frozen meal, for instance, can contain 50% or more of your daily sodium allowance. By replacing these foods with homemade alternatives, you regain control of your sodium intake.
3. ***Prioritize Calcium-Rich Foods***: Calcium is another nutrient that supports blood pressure regulation and reduces the impact of sodium. Dairy products like yogurt, fortified plant milks, or leafy greens like kale and broccoli are great sources to incorporate into your diet.
4. ***Monitor Your Blood Pressure***: Regularly check your blood pressure, either at home with a reliable device or during checkups with your doctor. Tracking trends over time can help you make timely adjustments to your diet and lifestyle.

Hidden Salt Triggers for Fatigue

Fatigue doesn't just stem from lack of sleep or physical exertion. For many, it's a result of their body being overburdened by excess sodium. When you consume large amounts of salt, your body holds onto water to dilute it and maintain balance. This water retention forces your heart and kidneys to work harder, which can leave you feeling tired and sluggish.

The sources of this excess sodium often aren't the obvious salty foods like chips or pretzels. Instead, it hides in processed and pre-packaged foods that you might not think twice about.

Where Sodium Hides in Your Diet

- *Breads and Baked Goods*: A single slice of bread can contain anywhere from 80–230 mg of sodium. This adds up quickly if you're eating sandwiches or breakfast pastries.
- *Canned Soups and Vegetables*: Many canned foods rely on sodium for preservation and flavor. Opt for low-sodium or no-salt-added versions when possible.
- *Condiments and Dressings*: Ketchup, soy sauce, salad dressings, and even hot sauces are packed with sodium. A tablespoon of soy sauce, for example, contains more than 1,000 mg of sodium. Choose low-sodium condiments or make your own at home.
- *Cheese and Processed Meats*: Foods like deli turkey, bacon, sausages, or even snack packs with cheese and crackers are sodium-heavy. Limiting these is key to maintaining your energy and managing salt intake.

Real-Life Strategies to Limit Hidden Sodium

1. *Check Nutrition Labels*: Look for sodium content on food packaging. A good rule of thumb is to aim for products with less than 140 mg of sodium per serving.

2. ***Be Mindful of Portion Sizes***: Even foods labeled "low-sodium" can add up if you're eating large quantities. Stick to recommended serving sizes.
3. ***DIY Seasonings and Dressings***: Replace store-bought dressings with DIY versions using olive oil, vinegar, mustard, and fresh herbs. For seasoning, experiment with spices like cumin, smoked paprika, or turmeric to replace salty flavors.
4. ***Cook More at Home***: Preparing meals from scratch allows you to control how much sodium you add. Batch cooking soups, sauces, or casseroles lets you avoid the high salt content of pre-made versions.

By addressing hidden sodium in your diet and making smarter food choices, you'll support your body's natural energy levels and avoid the fatigue that comes with a sodium-heavy routine.

By being mindful of sodium intake and taking practical steps, you can significantly reduce strain on your heart, maintain healthy blood pressure, and experience better energy and well-being overall. Small changes to what you eat and how you prepare your meals can have a lasting impact on your health as you move forward.

Where Salt Hides and How to Outsmart It

It's easy to think of salt as something you sprinkle from a shaker onto your plate. But a significant portion of the sodium in your diet is hidden in foods in ways you wouldn't expect. Even if you're cutting back on obviously salty snacks like chips or pretzels, sneaky sources of sodium could still be increasing your intake without your awareness.

Where Sodium Hides

1. *Processed and Packaged Foods*: Pre-made meals, frozen dinners, and instant soups often rely on high levels of sodium for flavor and preservation. A single frozen pizza or microwaveable pasta dish, for instance, can contain more than half your entire recommended daily sodium intake.
2. *Canned Vegetables and Soups*: While canned vegetables can be a convenient way to get more greens into your diet, they can also come packed in salty brine. Similarly, canned or instant soups are a common

source of hidden sodium; a single serving can contain 800 mg or more.
3. ***Condiments and Sauces***: Store-bought ketchup, soy sauce, barbecue sauce, and salad dressings often have a high sodium content. Shockingly, just one tablespoon of soy sauce can contain up to 900 mg of sodium.
4. ***Breads and Baked Goods***: Bread, muffins, and rolls don't taste overtly salty, but they can contribute heavily to daily sodium intake. A single slice of bread may have over 200 mg of sodium, which quickly adds up as part of a sandwich.
5. ***Cheeses and Deli Meats***: While they're convenient for snacks or sandwiches, deli meats, bacon, sausages, and processed cheeses are packed with sodium used in brining and curing processes.

How to Outsmart Hidden Sodium

1. ***Read Labels Religiously***: Many products, even healthy ones, hide sodium in their ingredient lists. Learning how to understand these labels will help reduce your intake (more on that below).
2. ***Choose Low- or No-Sodium Options***: Many canned goods, broths, and condiments have low-sodium or no-added-salt varieties. Opting for these can significantly cut your sodium without affecting flavor.
3. ***Rinse Before Use***: If you use canned beans or vegetables, drain and rinse them thoroughly under

running water. This can remove up to 40% of the sodium.
4. ***Cook from Scratch***: When possible, prepare meals at home using fresh ingredients. By cooking soups, sauces, or dressings yourself, you control how much salt gets added.
5. ***Season Creatively***: Trade salt for flavorful herbs and spices like garlic, paprika, pepper, or citrus zest. These seasonings add depth while keeping sodium levels in check.

Hidden sodium can sneak into your diet from unexpected sources, but small changes can make a big difference. By reading labels, choosing low-sodium options, and getting creative with seasoning, you can enjoy flavorful meals while keeping your sodium intake in check.

Common High-Sodium Foods at Home and Restaurants

Even if you think you're eating healthy, sodium can sneak into your diet in less obvious ways. Some of the most common high-sodium culprits are foods we eat regularly at home or order out when dining in restaurants.

At Home
1. ***Packaged Breakfast Cereals and Oatmeal***: Many cereals carry additional sodium for flavor. Even

flavored instant oatmeals can pack 200–250 mg or more per packet.
2. ***Crackers and Chips***: These snacks, while convenient, are often seasoned with large amounts of sodium. Even whole-grain versions can still be significant contributors to sodium intake.
3. ***Pasta Sauces and Jarred Foods***: A single serving of pasta sauce can contain up to 500 mg of sodium. Couple that with addition of grated cheese, and your sodium intake shoots up fast.
4. ***Frozen Vegetables with Sauce***: While plain frozen vegetables are a great choice, those with buttery or cheesy sauces frequently have added sodium.
5. ***Bouillon Cubes or Stock***: Soups or gravies made with bouillon or premade stock are often incredibly salty, even if the flavor profile doesn't seem overwhelming.

At Restaurants

1. ***Fast-Food Combo Meals***: Burgers, fries, and sodas are classic high-sodium offenders. While fries are visibly salty, buns alone are often surprisingly sodium-filled. The same goes for fried chicken sandwiches and salads with creamy dressings.
2. ***Chinese and Asian Cuisine***: Dishes using soy, teriyaki, or oyster sauce are typically very high in sodium. While these meals are flavorful, their salt content can be excessive.

3. ***Pizzas and Pasta Dishes***: While both are delicious, pizza crust, sauce, cheese, and toppings like pepperoni combine to create a major sodium bomb. Pasta dishes with jarred or pre-made sauces follow a similar pattern.
4. ***Chain Restaurant "Healthy" Entrees***: Grilled chicken, wraps, or low-calorie entrees may sound healthy but often rely on marinades, dressings, or seasonings packed with salt to amp up their flavor.

Hidden sodium is everywhere, from packaged snacks and sauces at home to fast food and restaurant dishes. Being mindful of these common sources can help you make healthier choices and reduce your overall sodium intake.

How to Read Nutrition Labels After 50 (Even Without Glasses!)

Nutrition labels can seem daunting, especially when dealing with small print or unfamiliar guidelines. But mastering these labels can be a game-changer for cutting back on sodium. Here are strategies to make it simple and practical.

Key Areas to Focus On

1. ***Serving Sizes***: Everything on the label is based on one serving size, so check how much of the product constitutes a single portion (e.g., one slice of bread versus two).

2. ***Sodium Content***: Sodium is often listed in milligrams (mg). Look for products that contain less than 140 mg per serving, which qualifies them as "low-sodium." If a product has more than 400 mg per serving, it's a high-sodium item and should be consumed sparingly.
3. ***Percent Daily Value (% DV)***: This tells you what percentage of your daily sodium intake the serving contributes. Aim to keep individual items closer to 5% rather than 20% or higher, especially if you plan to eat multiple servings in a day.
4. ***Ingredients List***: Look for high-sodium ingredients like salt, sodium chloride, monosodium glutamate (MSG), baking soda, or sodium-based preservatives closer to the beginning of the ingredients list (items are listed in order of quantity).

Label Terms and Their Meanings
- *"No Salt Added" or "Unsalted"*: These products haven't been salted during processing. However, they can still naturally contain sodium.
- *"Low-Sodium":* Products contain 140 mg of sodium or less per serving.
- *"Reduced Sodium"*: These products have 25% less sodium than the standard version but may still contain significant amounts.
- *"Sodium-Free"*: Items with fewer than 5 mg of sodium per serving.

Tricks to Make Reading Easier

1. *Carry Reading Glasses*: Even if they're just a small pair, stash them in your bag to avoid struggling with tiny text.
2. *Use Your Phone's Camera*: Snap a picture of labels and zoom in for a clearer, easier read.
3. *Focus on Key Sections*: When pressed for time, skip to sodium content, serving size, and % DV to make quick decisions.

Habits to Build Confidence

1. *Practice at Home*: Spend time comparing labels on products in your pantry. This makes it easier to spot healthier options when you're shopping in-store.
2. *Familiarize Yourself with Top Contenders*: Find and stick to low-sodium brands you trust so grocery trips are faster and less stressful.
3. *Make It a Routine*: Check labels regularly to build awareness of what you're consuming daily.

By learning to spot hidden sodium in your diet, recognizing high-sodium foods both at home and while dining out, and honing your skills with nutrition labels, you'll be better equipped to maintain heart health and manage your energy levels effectively.

What Happens When You Lower Sodium

Reducing sodium intake can have a profound impact on your overall health and well-being. From supporting your heart to boosting daily energy levels, cutting back on salt triggers multiple positive changes within your body. These benefits often begin to show within days and grow more noticeable over weeks and months. Here's a deeper look at what happens when you lower your sodium intake.

1. **Your Body Flushes Excess Water**

   When you consume too much sodium, your body retains extra water to maintain the proper balance in your cells. This water retention can lead to bloating, puffiness, and even weight fluctuations. By reducing sodium, your body starts to release the excess water, relieving bloating and helping you feel lighter overall.

2. **Blood Pressure Drops**

   One of the most immediate and critical benefits of lowering sodium is its impact on blood pressure.

Sodium causes blood vessels to constrict, increasing the volume of blood they need to accommodate and resulting in higher blood pressure. Switching to a lower-sodium diet helps relax these vessels, making it easier for your heart to pump blood and bringing your blood pressure down to healthier levels.

3. **Your Kidneys Get a Break**

   Your kidneys play a key role in processing sodium and maintaining fluid balance. A diet high in sodium places extra strain on these organs as they work overtime to flush out the excess. By reducing sodium intake, you ease this burden, supporting better kidney function and reducing your risk of long-term complications like kidney disease.

Heart Health Benefits

Below are some additional benefits of reducing your sodium intake for heart health:

1. **Reduced Risk of Cardiovascular Disease**

   High blood pressure is one of the leading risk factors for heart disease. A high-sodium diet forces your heart to work harder to pump blood, increasing strain on your arteries. Over time, this stress can lead to conditions such as heart attacks, strokes, and heart failure. By lowering sodium, you protect your heart and lower your risk of these potentially life-threatening issues. Studies show that even modest sodium reductions can make a significant difference in improving cardiovascular health outcomes.

2. **Less Vascular Stiffness**

   Sodium increases the workload on your blood vessels, causing them to become stiff and less elastic over time. This reduces their ability to adjust as needed to maintain proper circulation. A low-sodium diet helps prevent this stiffening, allowing your blood vessels to remain flexible and resilient. This contributes to better overall circulation and decreased risk of complications.

3. **Improved Cholesterol Levels**

   When you improve your eating habits to include more low-sodium, whole foods, you also tend to reduce your intake of processed foods. Many of these processed items are not just high in sodium but also in unhealthy trans fats. This shift toward healthier options can help lower bad cholesterol levels (LDL) and increase good cholesterol levels (HDL), further supporting your heart health.

Actionable Tip: To increase your heart-friendly nutrients, add foods like fatty fish, leafy greens, nuts, and seeds. These provide omega-3 fatty acids and potassium, which work in tandem with lower sodium to keep your heart in optimal shape.

Better Sleep, Less Bloating

Learn how cutting back on sodium can enhance your sleep, ease bloating, and support healthier digestion—helping you feel better, inside and out.

1. **Why Sodium Affects Sleep**

   High sodium levels can disrupt sleep patterns in a couple of surprising ways. Excess sodium causes fluid retention, which may increase blood pressure or result in nighttime interruptions like frequent urination. Additionally, salt-heavy meals close to bedtime can lead to indigestion, making it harder to fall and stay asleep.

   When you lower sodium in your diet, your body retains less water, reducing nighttime discomfort. You're likely to experience fewer mid-sleep trips to the bathroom and a more restful, uninterrupted sleep overall.

2. **Relief from Bloating**

   Bloating happens when your body holds onto excess water due to high sodium intake. This can lead to puffiness, especially in areas like your hands, feet, and face. By cutting back on salt, your body regulates its water levels more efficiently, minimizing bloating and helping you feel lighter and more comfortable.

Practical Example: Swelling in your ankles or fingers often decreases within a week of cutting back on sodium. Drinking plenty of water and eating diuretic-rich foods like cucumbers, celery, and watermelon can speed up the process.

3. **Digestive Benefits**

    A lower sodium diet tends to include more fiber-rich foods like fresh vegetables, legumes, and whole grains. These promote better digestion and reduce issues such as constipation or water retention, further easing abdominal bloating and discomfort.

Mood and Energy Boosts

Lowering your sodium intake doesn't just benefit your overall health—it can also boost your energy, improve your mood, and enhance your skin. Here's a detailed look at how reducing your sodium intake can have these positive effects on your body:

1. **Sodium's Impact on Energy Levels**

    When your body retains excess sodium, your heart and kidneys are forced to work harder, and this extra effort can drain your energy. High blood pressure caused by sodium may also leave you feeling fatigued or sluggish. Lowering your sodium intake helps reduce this physical strain, allowing your body to use energy more efficiently and leaving you feeling lighter and more energized.

2. **Stabilized Mood**

    Large sodium fluctuations can even impact mood regulation. When the body is under stress from excess sodium retention, it can contribute to feelings of irritability or brain fog. Lowering sodium may reduce general inflammation in the body, which has been linked to improved mood and mental clarity. Additionally, the increased nutrient density of low-sodium diets (more fresh fruits, vegetables, and healthy fats) provides vitamins and minerals like magnesium and potassium, which are critical for brain health.

3. **Clearer Skin**

    Dehydration caused by high sodium intake can lead to dull, dry skin and even contribute to swelling and puffiness in your face. By lowering sodium, you improve your body's ability to retain proper water levels, which benefits your skin's hydration, elasticity, and overall appearance.

Actionable Tips for Boosting Energy and Mood

1. ***Snack Smartly***: Swap salty snacks like pretzels or chips for energizing options like raw almonds, baby carrots with hummus, or fresh fruit. These provide longer-lasting energy without the energy crash.
2. ***Hydrate Consistently***: Drink plenty of water throughout the day to support sodium balance and prevent dehydration-related fatigue, especially after a salty meal.
3. ***Add Magnesium-Rich Foods***: Incorporate foods like dark chocolate, spinach, and nuts to improve mood and prevent fatigue. Magnesium plays an important role in relaxing muscles and calming the nervous system.

Lowering your sodium intake is not just about avoiding high blood pressure or protecting your heart, though those are key benefits. It's about setting yourself up to feel better every day. From sleeping soundly to feeling sharper and more energized, the small changes you make can ripple outward to improve every aspect of your health and well-being. By staying consistent, you can enjoy these lasting benefits and build habits that support vitality long into the future.

The 21-Day Action Plan for Lowering Sodium

Making long-term changes to reduce sodium in your diet doesn't have to feel overwhelming. This 21-day action plan breaks the process into manageable steps, guiding you through preparation, awareness, and implementation with easy tips, meal plans, and recipes. By the end of the three weeks, you'll be set up for success and already feeling the benefits of a healthier, low-sodium lifestyle.

Prep Week: Set Yourself Up for Success

Before you start making changes, it's important to prepare your kitchen, pantry, and mindset. Prep Week is all about getting organized and making the transition as seamless as possible.

Pantry Makeover

Take stock of your pantry, refrigerator, and freezer. Sodium often hides in processed, packaged, and seemingly innocent foods. Follow these steps for a complete pantry makeover.

- ***Identify Culprits***: Check the labels on canned goods, condiments, sauces, snacks, and pre-packaged mixes. Anything with "sodium" listed near the top of the ingredient list or more than 300 mg of sodium per serving is a red flag.
- ***Clear Out High-Sodium Foods***: Donate unopened, high-sodium items to a food bank or discard older products. Replace items like salty chips, pre-seasoned mixes, and jarred pasta sauces.
- ***Stock Up on Healthy Options***: Replace high-sodium foods with low-sodium or no-salt-added versions. Focus on whole ingredients like dried beans, unsalted nuts, frozen vegetables, and whole grains.

Easy Low-Sodium Substitutes

Transitioning to a lower-sodium diet doesn't mean giving up flavor. Here are simple swaps to cut sodium while keeping meals delicious.

- ***Trade Table Salt for Herbs and Spices***: Replace sodium with flavors such as garlic, cumin, paprika, or lemon zest. These add depth without the extra salt.
- ***Choose Low-Sodium Broths***: Use these for soups or grains like rice. You can also make your own broth using fresh vegetables, herbs, and water.
- ***Go Fresh Over Canned***: Opt for fresh or frozen vegetables instead of canned ones. If you must use

canned, rinse them thoroughly to remove excess sodium.
- *Swap Salty Snacks*: Replace chips or crackers with air-popped popcorn, unsalted nuts, or fruit slices.

Batch Cooking Tips

Cooking from scratch is one of the best ways to control sodium in your diet. Batch cooking ensures you have healthy, low-sodium meals ready throughout the week.

- *Plan a Cooking Day*: Dedicate a couple of hours to cooking in bulk for the week ahead.
- *Prepare Base Ingredients*: Cook large quantities of essentials like brown rice, quinoa, lentils, and grilled chicken. Store them in individual portions for easy access.
- *Make Freezer-Friendly Recipes*: Soups, stews, and casseroles freeze and reheat well. Use low-sodium ingredients to prepare these in advance.
- *Invest in Containers*: Store pre-cooked meals in airtight, portioned containers to save time while keeping food fresh.

Week 1: Awareness & Reset

Once your preparation is complete, it's time to focus on awareness. Week 1 is all about observing your habits and resetting your approach to meals.

What to Focus On

1. *Track Sodium Intake*: Use an app or a simple notebook to track what you eat and its sodium content. Pay attention to high-sodium foods and when you tend to consume them.
2. *Read Labels Carefully*: Check every label in your pantry and new grocery items. Look for products labeled "low-sodium" (140 mg or less per serving) or "no added salt."
3. *Drink Plenty of Water*: Staying hydrated helps flush out excess sodium from your system. Aim for at least 8 glasses a day.
4. *Break the Habit of Salting*: If you tend to sprinkle salt on everything, start using alternatives like pepper, vinegar, or fresh herbs instead.

7-Day Meal Plan for Week 1

Day 1

- *Breakfast*: Overnight oats made with unsalted almond milk, fresh blueberries, and a drizzle of honey.
- *Morning Snack*: Sliced cucumbers with 2 tbsp of low-sodium hummus.
- *Lunch*: Grilled chicken salad with spinach, cherry tomatoes, cucumber, and olive oil vinaigrette.
- *Afternoon Snack*: A small handful of unsalted almonds with an apple.

- **Dinner**: Baked salmon topped with lemon slices and dill, served with steamed broccoli and quinoa.

Day 2

- **Breakfast**: Scrambled eggs with fresh spinach, sautéed in olive oil on a slice of whole-grain toast.
- **Morning Snack**: A mix of unsalted trail mix (dried fruit, almonds, and pumpkin seeds).
- **Lunch**: Lentil soup made with low-sodium vegetable broth, paired with fresh apple slices.
- **Afternoon Snack**: Baby carrots and 1 tbsp of low-sodium peanut butter.
- **Dinner**: Turkey meatballs (made with whole-grain breadcrumbs and no-salt marinara) served over zucchini noodles.

Day 3

- **Breakfast**: Greek yogurt (unsweetened) topped with sliced bananas and a sprinkle of chia seeds.
- **Morning Snack**: Radish slices with 2 tbsp of avocado spread.
- **Lunch**: Grilled vegetable wrap with roasted zucchini, red peppers, and avocado spread on a whole-grain tortilla.
- **Afternoon Snack**: 1 orange and a handful of unsalted sunflower seeds.

- *Dinner*: Stir-fried tofu in sesame oil with snap peas, bell peppers, broccoli, and a drizzle of low-sodium soy sauce, served over brown rice.

Day 4

- *Breakfast*: Steel-cut oats cooked with unsweetened coconut milk, topped with raspberries and 1 tsp of shredded coconut.
- *Morning Snack*: A boiled egg with celery sticks.
- *Lunch*: Grilled chicken breast on a bed of arugula, mango slices, cucumber, and lime vinaigrette.
- *Afternoon Snack*: Cherry tomatoes with 1 oz of unsalted mozzarella cheese.
- *Dinner*: Herb-crusted baked cod with roasted sweet potatoes and asparagus.

Day 5

- *Breakfast*: A blend of spinach, frozen berries, unsweetened almond milk, and a tablespoon of chia seeds.
- *Morning Snack*: Homemade guacamole (mashed avocado with lime juice and cilantro) with bell pepper slices.
- *Lunch*: Asian-style grilled shrimp salad with mixed greens, shredded carrots, sesame oil, and a splash of rice vinegar.

- ***Afternoon Snack***: Handful of unsalted cashews with a pear.
- ***Dinner***: Spaghetti squash tossed with no-salt marinara, sautéed mushrooms, and a sprinkle of Parmesan.

Day 6

- ***Breakfast***: Cottage cheese (unsalted) with diced tomatoes and cracked black pepper, served with whole-grain crackers.
- ***Morning Snack***: Sliced strawberries with a dollop of Greek yogurt and a drizzle of honey.
- ***Lunch***: Lentil and spinach salad with diced cucumbers, cherry tomatoes, and olive oil vinaigrette.
- ***Afternoon Snack***: Sliced zucchini with 2 tbsp tahini dip.
- ***Dinner***: Grilled turkey burger (served on a whole-grain bun) with a side of baked sweet potato fries.

Day 7

- ***Breakfast***: Scrambled eggs with chopped bell peppers and onions, served with a side of orange slices.
- ***Morning Snack***: Rice cakes with 1 tbsp unsalted almond butter and a dash of cinnamon.
- ***Lunch***: Grilled chicken quinoa bowl with roasted zucchini, red onion, and a light lemon-tahini dressing.

- ***Afternoon Snack***: Frozen banana coins dipped in Greek yogurt (plain, unsweetened).
- ***Dinner***: Roasted vegetable medley (zucchini, carrots, and mushrooms) with grilled salmon and wild rice.

Follow these meals for a structured, beginner-friendly way to reset your eating habits, reduce sodium intake, and stay energized throughout the week.

Beginner-Friendly Recipes

Low-Sodium Lentil Soup

Ingredients:

- 1 cup lentils (rinsed)
- 4 cups low-sodium vegetable broth
- 1 cup chopped carrots
- 1 cup diced celery
- 1 small onion, diced
- 1 tsp cumin
- 1 bay leaf

Instructions:

1. Sauté onion, carrots, and celery in olive oil until softened.
2. Add lentils, broth, and spices. Bring to a boil.
3. Reduce heat and simmer for 30 minutes. Remove bay leaf and serve.

Baked Salmon with Lemon and Dill

Ingredients:

- 2 salmon fillets
- 1 lemon, sliced
- 1 tsp dried dill
- 1 tbsp olive oil

Instructions:

1. Preheat oven to 375°F.
2. Place salmon on a baking sheet lined with parchment paper. Drizzle with olive oil and sprinkle dill on top.
3. Lay lemon slices over the fish and bake for 15–20 minutes.

Shopping List

To make your low-sodium transition smoother, start your week with a well-prepared shopping list.

Produce:

- Fresh fruits (apples, bananas, oranges)
- Leafy greens (spinach, kale)
- Vegetables (zucchini, bell peppers, carrots, broccoli)

Proteins:

- Skinless chicken breasts
- Wild-caught salmon
- Tofu or tempeh

Pantry Items:

- Quinoa, brown rice, or couscous
- Unsalted nuts and seeds
- Low-sodium vegetable or chicken broth

Seasonings:

- Fresh garlic, dried herbs, and spices like paprika or black pepper
- Lemon or lime juice

By dividing the 21-day plan into manageable steps and equipping yourself with a variety of options, you'll be setting yourself up for success in reducing sodium and feeling better.

These steps allow you to build momentum, make lasting changes, and enjoy the noticeable benefits of a healthier, low-sodium life.

Week 2: Balance & Boost

Week 2 in your sodium-reduction plan is all about finding balance and boosting your efforts. Now that you've spent a week focusing on awareness and resetting your eating habits, it's time to build on that foundation. This week, you'll learn how to maintain your new habits in social settings, stay motivated when cooking for smaller households, and explore an updated 7-day meal plan with recipes and an easy shopping list.

How to Dine Out Smartly

Dining out doesn't mean you have to sacrifice your low-sodium goals. It just requires a little preparation and smart decision-making. Here's how to enjoy eating out while staying on track.

1. **Research Before You Go**

   Most restaurant menus are available online. Check the nutritional information, if possible, to find lower-sodium options ahead of time. Look for words like "grilled," "steamed," or "broiled," which usually indicate healthier choices, and avoid items labeled as "smoked," "cured," or "fried," as these tend to be higher in sodium.

2. **Make Special Requests**

Don't hesitate to ask for modifications. A few simple requests can make a big difference:

- Ask for sauces and dressings on the side to control how much you use.
- Request no added salt during cooking. Many chefs are happy to accommodate this.
- Opt for fresh, whole ingredients like grilled proteins and fresh vegetables over pre-seasoned options.

3. **Watch Out for Hidden Sodium**

Common culprits like bread, condiments, and side dishes often sneak in a lot of salt. Swap bread-based offerings for salad starters or vegetable sides, and skip high-sodium condiments like soy sauce or ketchup in favor of lemon wedges, olive oil, or a light vinaigrette.

Pro Tip: Save half your meal for later. Restaurant portions are often oversized, which means sodium levels are, too. Boxing up half for another day helps you eat less sodium all at once.

Staying Motivated When Cooking for One (or Two)

If you're cooking smaller portions, it's easy to lose motivation or feel like it's not worth the effort. But preparing meals at home is one of the best ways to control your sodium intake. Here's how to make cooking for one (or two) enjoyable and efficient.

1. *Simplify Your Recipes*: Stick to meals with just a few ingredients and minimal steps. Recipes like sheet-pan dinners or one-pot soups make cleanup a breeze while keeping sodium low.
2. *Utilize Leftovers*: Cook once, eat twice! Double your recipes and save leftovers for the next day's lunch or dinner. This reduces time spent cooking and eliminates the temptation to reach for processed meals.
3. *Invest in Freezer-Friendly Portions*: Batch cooking works well even for small households. Freeze individual portions of homemade soups, stews, or casseroles in airtight containers so you always have a healthy, low-sodium meal ready to go.
4. *Treat Cooking as Self-Care*: Shift your mindset. Think of cooking as a way to fuel your body, reduce stress, and care for yourself (or a loved one). Try experimenting with new herbs or spices to make it fun and create meals you genuinely look forward to eating.

Pro Tip: Make it social! Invite a friend or family member to join you for a meal. Sharing food makes the experience more enjoyable and motivates you to try new dishes.

7-Day Meal Plan for Week 2

Day 8

- *Breakfast*: Whole-grain avocado toast topped with sliced cherry tomatoes and a sprinkle of black pepper.
- *Morning Snack*: A small pear with a handful of unsalted walnuts.
- *Lunch*: Quinoa and black bean bowl with diced bell peppers, lime juice, and a sprinkle of cumin.
- *Afternoon Snack*: Baby cucumber slices with 2 tbsp of tahini dip.
- *Dinner*: Lemon-garlic grilled chicken breast with steamed green beans and roasted red potatoes.

Day 9

- *Breakfast*: Plain oatmeal cooked with unsalted almond milk, topped with chopped dates and a sprinkle of nutmeg.
- *Morning Snack*: Sliced celery sticks with no-salt-added peanut butter.
- *Lunch*: Mixed greens topped with grilled shrimp, mandarin oranges, sliced almonds, and balsamic vinaigrette.

- *Afternoon Snack*: A handful of unsalted seeds (like pumpkin or sunflower) with a few dried apricot pieces.
- *Dinner*: Baked cod with roasted asparagus and a side of whole-grain couscous.

Day 10

- *Breakfast*: A blend of unsweetened almond milk, spinach, frozen peaches, and a tablespoon of ground flaxseed.
- *Morning Snack*: A boiled egg with cherry tomatoes.
- *Lunch*: Turkey and avocado lettuce wraps with shredded carrots and a touch of mustard.
- *Afternoon Snack*: Apple slices with 1 tbsp unsalted almond butter.
- *Dinner*: Veggie stir-fry with tofu, broccoli, bell peppers, and mushrooms in sesame oil, served over wild rice.

Day 11

- *Breakfast*: Scrambled eggs with sautéed kale and a side of sliced cantaloupe.
- *Morning Snack*: Sliced cucumbers topped with 2 tbsp tuna salad (made with plain Greek yogurt).
- *Lunch*: Grilled chicken quinoa salad with cucumbers, red onion, and a light lemon vinaigrette.
- *Afternoon Snack*: Low-sodium popcorn seasoned with smoked paprika and garlic powder.

- ***Dinner***: Herb-baked salmon with roasted carrots and mashed sweet potatoes.

Day 12

- ***Breakfast***: Whole-grain English muffin with 1 tbsp unsalted almond butter and banana slices.
- ***Morning Snack***: Sliced bell peppers with guacamole.
- ***Lunch***: Lentil and kale soup with a side of whole-grain crackers.
- ***Afternoon Snack***: Greek yogurt (plain, unsweetened) with sliced strawberries and a drizzle of honey.
- ***Dinner***: Grilled turkey burger (on a lettuce wrap) with roasted Brussels sprouts and a baked potato topped with plain Greek yogurt.

Day 13

- ***Breakfast***: Avocado and egg breakfast bowl with diced tomatoes and a sprinkle of chili flakes.
- ***Morning Snack***: 1 orange with a handful of unsalted pistachios.
- ***Lunch***: Whole-grain pasta tossed with roasted zucchini, cherry tomatoes, and a drizzle of olive oil.
- ***Afternoon Snack***: Slices of pear served with 1 oz of unsalted cottage cheese.
- ***Dinner***: Baked chicken thighs with sautéed spinach and garlic, served with wild rice.

Day 14

- ***Breakfast***: Steel-cut oats cooked in unsweetened coconut milk, topped with diced apples and pumpkin seeds.
- ***Morning Snack***: Radish and cucumber slices with 2 tbsp no-salt-added hummus.
- ***Lunch***: Nicoise-inspired salad with baby greens, boiled egg, steamed green beans, and a drizzle of olive oil.
- ***Afternoon Snack***: A handful of unsalted trail mix with dried cranberries, almonds, and coconut flakes.
- ***Dinner***: Grilled tofu skewers with bell peppers, zucchini, and onion, served with a side of quinoa.

Follow this Week 2 meal plan to build on your progress from Week 1. The variety of meals and snacks will keep things exciting while helping you maintain a low-sodium, heart-healthy lifestyle.

Sample Recipes

Turkey and Avocado Wrap

Ingredients:

- 1 whole-grain tortilla
- 2 oz low-sodium turkey slices
- ¼ avocado, mashed
- A handful of spinach leaves
- Slices of tomato

Instructions:

1. Spread mashed avocado on the tortilla.
2. Layer turkey, spinach, and tomato slices.
3. Roll tightly, slice in half, and enjoy!

Grilled Chicken Stir-Fry

Ingredients:

- 1 chicken breast, sliced into strips
- 1 cup snap peas
- 1 cup shredded carrots
- 2 tbsp low-sodium soy sauce alternative
- 1 tbsp sesame oil

Instructions:

1. Heat sesame oil in a pan and cook chicken until golden brown.
2. Add vegetables and stir-fry for 5-7 minutes.
3. Drizzle with soy sauce alternative and serve over brown rice.

Shopping List

Plan ahead with this comprehensive shopping list for the week.

Produce:

- Leafy greens (spinach, mixed greens)
- Fresh fruits (strawberries, blueberries, apples, bananas)
- Vegetables (carrots, snap peas, asparagus, cucumbers, cherry tomatoes)

Proteins:

- Chicken breast
- Cod fillets
- Ground turkey

Grains & Legumes:

- Low-sodium whole-grain bread or tortillas
- Quinoa
- Brown rice
- Lentils

Pantry Staples:

- Olive oil
- Low-sodium soy sauce alternative
- Herbs and spices (paprika, dill, garlic powder, cumin)
- Unsweetened almond milk

Extras:

- Greek yogurt (plain, unsweetened)
- Unsalted nuts for snacks
- Low-sodium granola

By following this plan, you'll strike a perfect balance between maintaining low-sodium habits and enjoying meals that fuel your energy. It's all about keeping things simple yet flavorful, and proving to yourself that a healthier lifestyle can be both practical and satisfying.

Week 3: Lasting Habits

After two weeks of resetting and balancing your sodium intake, Week 3 is about creating habits that last. The goal this week is to ensure the changes you've made become part of your everyday life. By learning how to spot hidden salt, using flavorful substitutes, and sticking to your meal plan, you'll confidently maintain your low-sodium lifestyle.

How to Spot Hidden Salt in "Healthy" Foods

Not all foods labeled "healthy" are low in sodium. Many options marketed as better-for-you alternatives are surprisingly salty. Here's how to uncover the hidden sodium in your grocery store.

1. **Read Beyond the Label**: Buzzwords like "organic," "natural," or "gluten-free" don't automatically mean

low sodium. Flip the package over and check the nutrition label.
- ***Look at Serving Size***: A single serving might not seem high in sodium, but if the portion size is small, the overall sodium content adds up quickly.
- ***Sodium Per Serving***: Aim for foods with less than 140 mg of sodium per serving, which is considered low-sodium by FDA standards.
- ***Check Ingredients List***: Sodium can sneak in under names like monosodium glutamate (MSG), sodium benzoate, or baking soda.

2. **Beware of Processed "Health" Foods**: Even foods marketed as healthy can be sodium traps. Be cautious with these common culprits:
   - ***Plant-Based Meats***: Many vegetarian or vegan meat substitutes contain high levels of sodium to mimic flavor.
   - ***Protein or Energy Bars***: Certain bars can pack in 200–300 mg of sodium for a small snack. Look for low-sodium options instead.
   - ***Canned Soups and Vegetables***: Choose "no salt added" varieties or rinse regular canned vegetables thoroughly.

Pro Tip: Prioritize whole foods like fresh fruits, vegetables, lean proteins, and grains. Whole foods naturally contain less sodium than anything processed or pre-packaged.

Flavor Without Salt: Herbs, Citrus & Smart Fats

One of the most exciting parts of reducing sodium is discovering creative ways to flavor your food. You'll quickly realize that salt isn't necessary for delicious meals!

1. **Boost Flavor with Herbs and Spices:** Herbs and spices add depth to your food while allowing you to skip the salt shaker.
    - *Fresh Herbs*: Basil, cilantro, parsley, dill, and rosemary can brighten up any dish.
    - *Spices*: Add cumin, turmeric, smoked paprika, or black pepper to soups, stews, and rubs for bold, savory flavors.
    - *Blends*: Create your own salt-free seasoning mix with garlic powder, onion powder, oregano, thyme, and paprika.
2. **Use Citrus for a Punch of Freshness:** Lemon and lime juice are fantastic for adding tangy brightness to your meals.
    - *Marinades*: Use them as a base for marinades with olive oil and garlic.
    - *Finishing Touches*: Squeeze fresh lemon over roasted vegetables, fish, chicken, or salads to enhance the natural flavors.
3. **Add Smart Fats for Richness:** Healthy fats give meals a satisfying, creamy texture without the need for salt.

- *Avocado*: Mash it onto toast or slice it into salads for a buttery flavor.
- *Nuts and Seeds*: Unsalted almonds, walnuts, or sunflower seeds add crunch and richness.
- *Olive Oil*: Drizzle extra-virgin olive oil onto finished dishes for a silky finish and robust taste.

Pro Tip: Experiment! Cooking with low sodium encourages creativity. Try combinations of your favorite herbs, spices, and citrus to find new go-to flavors.

7-Day Sample Meal Plan for Week 3

Day 15

Breakfast: Spinach and mushroom omelette with a small slice of whole-grain toast.

Morning Snack: Unsalted trail mix made with almonds, walnuts, raisins, and dried cranberries.

Lunch: Grilled chicken quinoa bowl with cucumbers, cherry tomatoes, and a lemon vinaigrette.

Afternoon Snack: Sliced carrots and celery with 2 tbsp no-salt-added hummus.

Dinner: Garlic-roasted cod with sautéed green beans and a side of brown rice.

Day 16

Breakfast: Overnight oats made with unsweetened almond milk, cinnamon, and fresh apple chunks.

Morning Snack: Greek yogurt (plain, unsweetened) topped with a handful of blueberries and 1 tsp chia seeds.

Lunch: Lentil and kale soup served with half an avocado on whole-grain bread.

Afternoon Snack: A small orange with a handful of unsalted sunflower seeds.

Dinner: Veggie-packed turkey chili with a side of roasted sweet potato wedges.

Day 17

Breakfast: Greek yogurt parfait layered with unsalted granola, sliced bananas, and raspberries.

Morning Snack: Sliced bell peppers with mashed avocado.

Lunch: Turkey and spinach wrap in a whole-grain tortilla with Dijon mustard.

Afternoon Snack: Sliced pear with 1 tbsp unsalted almond butter.

Dinner: Grilled salmon served with roasted Brussels sprouts and mashed cauliflower.

Day 18

Breakfast: Steel-cut oats cooked with unsweetened coconut milk, topped with diced mango and a sprinkle of nutmeg.

Morning Snack: A boiled egg with a handful of cherry tomatoes.

Lunch: Mixed green salad with sliced grilled chicken breast, cucumbers, orange segments, and balsamic vinaigrette.

Afternoon Snack: Cucumber slices with 2 tbsp tahini dip.

Dinner: Herb-roasted chicken thighs with steamed broccoli and wild rice.

Day 19

Breakfast: Whole-grain avocado toast with a sprinkle of cumin and sliced radishes.

Morning Snack: Handful of unsalted cashews with a small apple.

Lunch: Lentil and spinach stew with a side of roasted zucchini rounds.

Afternoon Snack: Radishes and cucumber slices with plain Greek yogurt for dipping.

Dinner: Baked cod topped with lemon slices and parsley, served with sautéed asparagus and quinoa.

Day 20

Breakfast: Scrambled eggs with sautéed kale, red bell peppers, and a side of cantaloupe slices.

Morning Snack: Rice cakes with 1 tbsp unsalted almond butter and banana slices.

Lunch: Quinoa salad with avocado, cherry tomatoes, cucumbers, and a light olive oil dressing.

Afternoon Snack: A boiled egg served with sliced carrots.

Dinner: Tofu stir-fry with broccoli, snap peas, and carrots over brown rice, seasoned with low-sodium soy sauce.

Day 21

Breakfast: A combination of unsweetened almond milk, spinach, frozen mixed berries, and a tablespoon of ground flaxseed.

Morning Snack: Handful of unsalted pistachios and a small orange.

Lunch: Nicoise-inspired salad with baby greens, boiled egg, steamed green beans, and a drizzle of olive oil.

Afternoon Snack: Sliced cucumber and celery with 2 tbsp no-salt-added hummus.

Dinner: Grilled shrimp skewers with bell peppers, zucchini, and onion, served with a wild rice pilaf.

Sample Recipes

Garlic-Roasted Cod

Ingredients:

- 2 cod fillets
- 2 cloves garlic, minced
- 1 tbsp olive oil
- Zest of 1 lemon
- 1 tsp dried parsley

Instructions:

1. Preheat oven to 375°F.
2. Place cod fillets on a baking sheet and rub with garlic, olive oil, and lemon zest.
3. Sprinkle parsley over the top and roast for 15–20 minutes until flaky.

Veggie-Packed Turkey Chili

Ingredients:

- 1 lb ground turkey
- 1 cup chopped bell peppers
- 1 cup diced zucchini
- 1 can no-salt-added diced tomatoes
- 2 cups low-sodium chicken broth
- 2 tsp cumin
- 1 tsp smoked paprika

Instructions:

1. Sauté turkey until browned. Add peppers and zucchini, cooking until softened.
2. Stir in spices, tomatoes, and broth. Simmer for 30 minutes, stirring occasionally.

Shopping List

Stocking up on the right ingredients at the start of the week can save time and stress.

Produce:

- Fresh herbs (cilantro, parsley, dill)
- Fresh fruits (apples, lemons, limes, berries)
- Vegetables (spinach, mushrooms, zucchini, bell peppers)

Proteins:

- Cod fillets
- Ground turkey
- Chicken breast

Grains & Legumes:

- Quinoa
- Brown rice
- Lentils

Pantry Staples:

- No-salt-added broth or diced tomatoes
- Olive oil
- Unsalted nuts

Seasonings:

Garlic, cumin, paprika, onion powder, parsley

Finish Week 3 strong by consistently practicing these strategies. Solidify your habits, experiment with flavors, and rely on your plan to create an effortless routine. Soon, eating low-sodium won't feel like a challenge; it'll become second nature!

Low-Sodium Recipe Toolkit

Cooking heart-healthy, low-sodium meals doesn't have to be bland or overwhelming. With the right ingredients and some creative techniques, you can enjoy meals that are packed with flavor while supporting your heart and energy levels. This Low-Sodium Recipe Toolkit offers simple, practical recipes designed to fit your lifestyle and tastes.

Comfort Foods Made Heart-Healthy

Low-Sodium Shepherd's Pie

Serves: 6

Ingredients:

- 1 lb lean ground turkey or beef
- 1 cup no-salt-added chicken broth
- 2 cups mixed vegetables (peas, carrots, green beans)
- 4 medium potatoes, peeled and cubed
- 2 tbsp olive oil or unsalted butter
- ½ cup unsweetened almond milk
- 1 tsp garlic powder

Instructions:

1. Preheat your oven to 375°F (190°C).
2. Boil the potatoes in salted water for 15-20 minutes or until fork-tender. Drain and mash with olive oil, almond milk, and garlic powder. Set aside.
3. While the potatoes cook, heat a skillet over medium heat. Add the ground turkey or beef and cook until browned.
4. Add the vegetables and chicken broth to the skillet. Cook until the broth has mostly evaporated and vegetables are tender, about 5-7 minutes.

5. Spread the meat and veggie mixture evenly in a baking dish. Layer the mashed potatoes on top, smoothing with a spoon or spatula.
6. Bake in the preheated oven for 20-25 minutes, or until the top turns a light golden brown.

Low-Sodium Vegetable Lasagna

Serves: 6

Ingredients:

- 12 no-boil whole grain lasagna noodles
- 1 jar no-salt-added marinara sauce
- 2 cups ricotta cheese (low-sodium)
- 2 cups fresh spinach, chopped
- 2 cups shredded mozzarella cheese (low-sodium)
- 1 small zucchini, thinly sliced

Instructions:

1. Preheat your oven to 375°F (190°C).
2. Mix ricotta cheese and spinach in a bowl. Season with black pepper if desired.
3. Spread a thin layer of marinara sauce along the bottom of a 9x13 baking dish.
4. Layer noodles, ricotta-spinach mixture, zucchini slices, marinara sauce, and mozzarella cheese. Repeat layers until ingredients are used up, ending with mozzarella on top.
5. Cover the dish with foil and bake for 25 minutes.
6. Remove the foil and bake for an additional 10 minutes to slightly brown the cheese.

Low-Sodium Sloppy Joes

Serves: 4

Ingredients:

- 1 lb lean ground beef or turkey
- 1 cup no-salt-added tomato sauce
- 1 tbsp apple cider vinegar
- 1 tbsp honey
- 1 tsp smoked paprika
- 4 whole-grain buns

Instructions:

1. Heat a skillet over medium heat. Add the ground beef or turkey and cook until browned, breaking it up into crumbles as it cooks.
2. Stir in the tomato sauce, apple cider vinegar, honey, and smoked paprika. Simmer for 10 minutes, allowing the flavors to meld.
3. Toast the whole-grain buns lightly and spoon the Sloppy Joe mixture onto each bun.
4. Serve with a side of mixed greens or carrot sticks.

Low-Sodium Chicken Alfredo

Serves: 4

Ingredients:

- 12 oz whole-grain fettuccine or pasta
- 1 tbsp olive oil
- 1 tbsp whole-wheat flour
- 1 ½ cups unsalted almond milk
- ½ cup grated Parmesan cheese
- 1 cup cooked shredded chicken

Instructions:

1. Prepare fettuccine according to package instructions. Reserve ½ cup of pasta water, then drain the remaining water.
2. Heat olive oil in a saucepan on medium heat. Stir in the flour to form a paste. Slowly whisk in almond milk, stirring constantly to avoid lumps.
3. Once the mixture thickens, stir in Parmesan cheese until fully melted. If the sauce is too thick, add a small amount of reserved pasta water.
4. Combine the sauce with cooked pasta and shredded chicken. Serve immediately.

Heart-Healthy Mashed Potato Bowl

Serves: 4

Ingredients:

- 4 cups prepared mashed potatoes (made with no-sodium broth or unsalted butter)
- 1 cup steamed broccoli florets
- 1 cup shredded cooked chicken or turkey
- 1 cup no-salt-added gravy

Instructions:

1. Warm the mashed potatoes and spoon them into individual serving bowls.
2. Top each bowl with a layer of steamed broccoli florets and shredded chicken.
3. Pour warm gravy evenly over each portion and serve immediately.

Quick Lunches for Energy

Zesty Quinoa Salad

Serves: 2

Ingredients:

- 1 cup cooked quinoa
- ½ cup corn kernels (fresh or unsalted)
- ½ cup black beans, rinsed
- 1 tbsp lime juice
- 1 tbsp olive oil
- ½ tsp chili powder
- 2 tbsp chopped cilantro

Instructions:

1. Combine the quinoa, corn, and black beans in a large bowl.
2. Whisk together lime juice, olive oil, chili powder, and cilantro in a small bowl.
3. Pour the dressing over the quinoa mixture and toss gently until evenly coated.
4. Serve chilled or at room temperature for a fresh, tangy lunch.

Turkey and Avocado Wrap

Serves: 2

Ingredients:

- 4 slices low-sodium turkey
- 2 whole-grain tortillas
- 1 avocado, mashed
- 1 cup spinach leaves
- 1 tbsp Dijon mustard (low-sodium)

Instructions:

1. Spread mashed avocado evenly over the tortillas.
2. Layer each tortilla with turkey and spinach leaves.
3. Drizzle a small amount of Dijon mustard over the fillings.
4. Roll the tortillas tightly, slice in half, and enjoy.

Low-Sodium Tuna Salad

Serves: 2

Ingredients:

- 1 can tuna in water, drained (low-sodium)
- 2 tbsp Greek yogurt
- ½ tsp Dijon mustard
- 1 celery stalk, chopped
- 1 tsp lemon juice

Instructions:

1. Combine the tuna, Greek yogurt, Dijon mustard, celery, and lemon juice in a bowl. Mix well.
2. Serve on whole-grain toast as a sandwich or over mixed greens as a salad.

Caprese Salad with a Twist

Serves: 2

Ingredients:

- 2 medium tomatoes, sliced
- 1 ball fresh mozzarella (low-sodium), sliced
- Fresh basil leaves
- 1 tbsp balsamic vinegar
- 1 tsp olive oil

Instructions:

1. Arrange the tomato slices, mozzarella, and basil leaves on a plate in alternating layers.
2. Drizzle with balsamic vinegar and olive oil.
3. Serve immediately as a light, refreshing lunch option.

Egg Salad Wrap

Serves: 2

Ingredients:

- 4 boiled eggs, chopped
- 2 tbsp Greek yogurt
- 1 tsp paprika
- 1 scallion, finely chopped
- 2 whole-grain tortillas

Instructions:

1. Mix chopped eggs, Greek yogurt, paprika, and scallions in a bowl until well combined.
2. Spread the egg salad evenly over the tortillas.
3. Roll the tortillas tightly, slice them in half, and serve.

Batch Dinners for the Week

Stuffed Bell Peppers

Serves: 4

Ingredients:

- 4 large bell peppers, halved and deseeded
- 1 cup cooked quinoa
- 1 cup no-salt-added marinara sauce
- ½ cup shredded low-sodium cheese
- ½ cup black beans

Instructions:

1. Preheat the oven to 375°F (190°C).
2. Mix the quinoa, marinara sauce, and black beans in a bowl.
3. Fill each bell pepper half with the quinoa mixture.
4. Arrange in a baking dish, cover with foil, and bake for 25 minutes.
5. Remove the foil, sprinkle with cheese, and bake for another 10 minutes.

Vegetable Stir-Fry

Serves: 4

Ingredients:

- 2 cups broccoli florets
- 1 cup sliced carrots
- 1 cup snap peas
- 1 red bell pepper, sliced
- 2 tbsp low-sodium soy sauce
- 1 tbsp sesame oil
- 1 tsp minced ginger

Instructions:

1. Heat sesame oil in a large pan over medium-high heat. Add ginger and sauté for 1 minute.
2. Add the vegetables and stir-fry for 5-7 minutes, until tender yet crisp.
3. Drizzle the soy sauce over the veggies, toss to combine, and serve.

Slow Cooker Lentil Soup

Serves: 6

Ingredients:

- 1 cup lentils, rinsed
- 4 cups low-sodium vegetable broth
- 1 cup chopped carrots
- 1 cup chopped celery
- 1 tsp cumin
- 1 tsp smoked paprika

Instructions:

1. Place all ingredients in a slow cooker.
2. Cook on low for 6 hours or on high for 3 hours, until the lentils are tender.
3. Serve warm with a small sprinkle of fresh parsley if desired.

Greek-Style Chicken Bowls

Serves: 4

Ingredients:

- 2 cups cooked brown rice
- 1 cup grilled, sliced chicken breast
- 1 cup chopped cucumber
- ½ cup crumbled feta (optional - use low-sodium)
- 1 tbsp olive oil
- 1 tbsp lemon juice

Instructions:

1. Divide brown rice into four bowls.
2. Top each bowl with chicken, cucumber, and feta.
3. Drizzle olive oil and lemon juice over the bowl before serving.

Turkey Meatballs in Tomato Sauce

Serves: 4

Ingredients:

- 1 lb ground turkey
- 1 egg
- ¼ cup whole-wheat breadcrumbs
- ½ tsp garlic powder
- 1 jar no-salt-added marinara sauce

Instructions:

1. Mix turkey, egg, breadcrumbs, and garlic powder in a bowl. Form into small meatballs.
2. Heat a large skillet over medium heat and brown the meatballs on all sides.
3. Pour the marinara sauce over the meatballs, cover, and simmer for 15 minutes.

Flavorful Dressings & Seasonings

Orange-Tahini Dressing

Ingredients:

- 2 tbsp tahini
- 1 tbsp fresh orange juice
- 1 tsp olive oil

Instructions:

1. Add tahini, orange juice, and olive oil to a small bowl.
2. Whisk until the mixture is smooth and creamy.
3. Drizzle over salads, grain bowls, or roasted vegetables.

Garlic Herb Vinaigrette

Ingredients:

- 2 tbsp olive oil
- 1 tbsp red wine vinegar
- 1 garlic clove, minced
- 1 tsp dried oregano
- ½ tsp Dijon mustard (optional for thickness)

Instructions:

1. Combine olive oil, vinegar, garlic, oregano, and Dijon mustard in a small jar with a lid.
2. Shake well until all ingredients are emulsified.
3. Use immediately or store in the fridge for up to one week.

Coconut Lime Dressing

Ingredients:

- 2 tbsp light coconut milk
- 1 tbsp lime juice
- 1 tsp honey
- ½ tsp grated fresh ginger

Instructions:

1. Whisk together coconut milk, lime juice, honey, and ginger in a small bowl.
2. Pour over mixed greens, grilled chicken, or shrimp.

Smoky Paprika Rub

Ingredients:

- 1 tsp smoked paprika
- ½ tsp garlic powder
- ½ tsp onion powder
- 1 tsp ground cumin

Instructions:

1. Combine all the spices in a small container. Mix thoroughly.
2. Rub onto chicken, fish, or tofu before grilling, roasting, or baking.

Lemon-Dill Marinade

Ingredients:

- 2 tbsp olive oil
- 1 tbsp lemon juice
- 1 tsp fresh dill, finely chopped
- ½ tsp black pepper

Instructions:

1. Combine olive oil, lemon juice, dill, and black pepper in a bowl. Stir well.
2. Use as a marinade for salmon, chicken, or veggies. Marinate for at least 30 minutes before cooking.

Guilt-Free Snacks

Carrot Sticks and Hummus

Ingredients:

- 4 medium carrots, peeled and cut into sticks
- 1 cup homemade or store-bought no-salt-added hummus

Instructions:

1. Peel and cut the carrots into snack-sized sticks.
2. Serve with a portion of hummus for dipping.

Nut-Free Energy Bites

Ingredients:

- 1 cup rolled oats
- ¼ cup sunflower seed butter
- 2 tbsp honey
- 2 tbsp chia seeds

Instructions:

1. Combine oats, sunflower seed butter, honey, and chia seeds in a large bowl. Stir until evenly mixed.
2. Roll the mixture into bite-sized balls (about 1 tbsp each).
3. Chill in the refrigerator for 30 minutes before serving.

Baked Sweet Potato Chips

Ingredients:

- 2 medium sweet potatoes, thinly sliced
- 1 tbsp olive oil
- ½ tsp smoked paprika

Instructions:

1. Preheat oven to 375°F (190°C). Line a baking sheet with parchment paper.
2. Toss sweet potato slices with olive oil and smoked paprika.
3. Spread slices in a single layer on the prepared baking sheet.
4. Bake for 20-25 minutes, flipping halfway through, until crispy.

Frozen Banana Coins

Ingredients:

- 2 ripe bananas, sliced into coins
- ½ cup unsweetened Greek yogurt
- 2 tbsp finely chopped unsalted nuts (optional)

Instructions:

1. Dip banana slices into Greek yogurt, coating all sides.
2. Place the slices on a parchment-lined tray and sprinkle with chopped nuts if desired.
3. Freeze for at least 2 hours before serving.

Apple Nachos

Ingredients:

- 1 large apple, thinly sliced
- 1 tbsp almond butter (unsalted)
- 1 tbsp unsalted granola
- 1 tsp honey

Instructions:

1. Arrange apple slices in a single layer on a plate.
2. Drizzle almond butter and honey over the apple slices.
3. Sprinkle with granola.

With these flavorful dressings, seasonings, and guilt-free snacks, you can bring variety and excitement to your low-sodium diet, making it easier to maintain heart health and energy while enjoying every bite!

Maintaining a Low-Sodium, Heart-Healthy Lifestyle

Transitioning to a low-sodium, heart-healthy diet can feel like a big change at first, but the key to sustaining it is finding approaches that fit your life. This section offers practical strategies and real-world solutions to help women over 50 stick with their goals beyond the initial 21 days, even when life gets busy or challenging.

How to Keep It Up After 21 Days

The 21-day mark is a significant milestone on your healthy eating journey. Here's how to stay on track as you move beyond this critical point:

1. *Celebrate Your Wins*: Reflect on what you've achieved so far, whether it's trying new recipes, noticing more energy, or improving your heart health. Celebrate these small victories to stay motivated.
2. *Build a Routine*: Establish consistency by planning meals at the same time each week. A Sunday meal

prep session or setting aside time to grocery shop can help you stick with your low-sodium plan.
3. ***Experiment with Flavors***: Boredom can derail progress. Keep it exciting by trying new herbs, spices, or recipes monthly. Cooking low-sodium meals doesn't have to mean sacrificing taste.
4. ***Focus on Your Goals***: Remind yourself of why you started. Whether it's supporting your heart health, enjoying more time with family, or feeling better day-to-day, your "why" is your anchor.
5. ***Allow Flexibility***: Perfection isn't necessary. A higher-sodium meal on occasion won't undo your progress. Focus on consistency, not rigidity.

Quick Tip: Keep your kitchen stocked with staples like fresh produce, lean proteins, and easy snacks to prevent decisions that derail plans.

When You Don't Feel Like Cooking

Cooking every day isn't always realistic, and that's okay. Here's how to stick with your heart-healthy goals even on days when motivation is low.

- ***Batch Cooking is a Lifesaver***: Prep meals in advance during your high-energy days and freeze portions for later. Having healthy options ready to warm up can turn a lazy evening into an easy success.

- *Opt for No-Cook Meals*: Assemble quick bites like salads, wraps, or veggie and hummus platters that require little to no preparation.
- *Choose Quality Convenience Foods*: Keep no-salt-added soups, frozen veggies, or pre-cooked quinoa and chicken on hand for effortless meals.
- *Invite Help*: If you live with others, ask family members to help cook or take over for the night. Sharing the load can make all the difference.

Energy-Saving Strategy: Use kitchen gadgets like a slow cooker, Instant Pot, or air fryer for nearly hands-free meal prep.

Handling Parties, Travel & Family Pressure

Social settings and busy schedules don't have to disrupt your progress. Here's how to manage these situations while staying true to your goals.

1. **Navigate Parties with Confidence**
   - *Bring Your Own Dish*: Contribute a low-sodium option like a fresh salad, veggie platter, or your favorite heart-healthy side dish.
   - *Choose Wisely*: Fill your plate with whole foods like fruits, veggies, and lean proteins. Limit sauces, dressings, and salty snacks.

2. **Stay Prepared During Travel**
   - Pack snacks like unsalted nuts, low-sodium crackers, or individual hummus cups for trips.
   - Research restaurant menus in advance and opt for grilled or steamed dishes when eating out. Politely request sauces and dressings on the side.
3. **Respond to Family Pressure**
   - Kindly explain your goals and educate loved ones about your low-sodium choices.
   - Suggest recipes enhanced with vibrant herbs and spices so everyone can enjoy flavorful meals together.

Social Tip: Practice mindful eating. Focus on the company and conversation instead of the food to help you stay present and intentional during gatherings.

Real-Life Maintenance Plan

Sustaining a heart-healthy, low-sodium lifestyle for the long term is easier with a practical plan. Here's how to make it work seamlessly in your life.

1. *Set Realistic Goals*: Aim to hit your daily sodium target most of the time rather than all the time. This approach is less stressful and more sustainable.
2. *Track Progress and Adjust*: Keep a food journal or use an app to track your meals and sodium intake. Adjust

your approach as needed based on what works best for your routine.
3. ***Schedule Regular Check-Ins***: Periodically review your goals and progress. Celebrate milestones like eating out successfully or trying five new recipes in a month.
4. ***Reconnect with Support***: Join local or online groups focused on low-sodium living for shared encouragement and accountability. Scheduling check-ins with a dietitian can also keep you on track.
5. ***Prioritize Enjoyment***: A sustainable lifestyle is one you enjoy. Experiment with new recipes, take a cooking class, or explore farmers' markets to keep it exciting.

Pro-Tip: Keep a list of your favorite low-sodium recipes, sauces, and snacks handy for inspiration when planning your week.

These strategies are designed to fit your real life, helping you manage heart health, stay energized, and keep your low-sodium lifestyle both practical and enjoyable for years to come.

Conclusion

Making the shift to a low-sodium lifestyle has extraordinary benefits that extend far beyond the kitchen. You've gained a deep understanding of why paying attention to sodium matters, especially after 50, and you now have the resources and knowledge to manage it with ease. This journey is not just about reducing salt; it's about gaining more control over your health, energy levels, and overall vitality. With every small change you make, you're creating a stronger foundation for a satisfying, heart-healthy life.

What's truly empowering is how achievable this transformation is. By prioritizing whole foods, seasoning dishes with vibrant herbs and spices, and spotting hidden sodium in packaged goods, you've equipped yourself with the tools you need to stay consistent. You've shown yourself that flavor doesn't depend on salt. Instead, simple swaps like using lemon juice or roasted garlic have opened new doors, making each meal a delightful experience. These strategies, once seemingly small, collectively reshape your approach to food.

The benefits of lowering sodium are felt in every part of your life. From reduced bloating and increased energy to better heart health and improved sleep, each positive outcome makes it clear that these changes are worth it. You've probably noticed that cooking at home no longer feels like a chore but an opportunity to explore creative, nutritious meals. Batch cooking, freezer-friendly recipes, and efficient meal prep ensure your efforts go further, leaving you more time to focus on what matters most in your day-to-day life.

Another significant win is how adaptable this lifestyle is to your routine. Even when presented with challenges like dining out, travel, or hosting a gathering, you've learned to make thoughtful, informed choices that align with your goals. Simple adjustments, like selecting grilled options or keeping sauces on the side, show that flexibility and progress can go hand in hand. It's these sustainable practices that pave the way for long-term success.

The shift you've embraced is less about restriction and more about empowerment. You're taking charge of your health while enjoying flavorful meals, feeling better, and gaining control over factors that once seemed out of reach. By mastering these new habits, you've cultivated a lifestyle that supports not only your body but also your confidence and peace of mind.

The effort you've put into adjusting your diet has been a worthwhile investment. With consistent, thoughtful changes, you're now equipped to maintain this lifestyle effortlessly. The steps you've taken so far are achievements that should fill you with pride. By reducing sodium and prioritizing heart-healthy choices, you've given yourself a gift that keeps on giving.

Every flavorful dish you prepare and every informed decision you make brings you closer to sustaining these changes for the long term. The vibrant, energetic you that's emerging is proof that small, intentional steps lead to lasting results. With your foundation firmly in place, you're on a path to not only healthier living but also greater enjoyment in all aspects of your life. Keep building on this success, and continue thriving every step of the way.

FAQs

How do I transition into a low-sodium diet without feeling overwhelmed?

Start with small changes instead of an immediate overhaul. Focus on replacing high-sodium foods with low-sodium options like fresh vegetables, whole grains, and lean proteins. Experiment with herbs, citrus, and spices to add flavor, and aim to prepare more meals at home where you control the ingredients.

What are some simple ways to add flavor to food without using salt?

Use fresh herbs like basil, rosemary, and cilantro, or spices like smoked paprika, cumin, and turmeric for bold flavors. Lemon and lime juice add brightness, while ingredients like garlic or ginger give dishes depth. You can also try olive oil drizzles or unsalted nuts for richness.

How can I enjoy eating out while keeping my sodium intake in check?

Check menus ahead of time and look for grilled or steamed dishes. Request sauces and dressings on the side and ask for no added salt during preparation. Choosing fresh options like salads or simply seasoned proteins can help you stick to low-sodium goals while dining out.

How do I handle family or friends who might not understand my low-sodium lifestyle?

Be open about your goals and explain how reducing sodium benefits your health. Offer to prepare or bring a flavorful low-sodium dish to share. Showing that healthy meals can still be delicious might even inspire others to try them.

Are there quick, low-sodium snack options for busy days?

Absolutely! Try snacks like fresh fruit, unsalted nuts, sliced veggies with hummus, or rice cakes with almond butter. Homemade trail mix made from unsweetened dried fruit and seeds is another convenient option.

What should I keep in my pantry to stay prepared for a low-sodium diet?

Stock up on essentials like no-salt-added broths, canned beans, and sauces; whole grains like quinoa and brown rice; herbs and spices; unsalted nuts; and fresh or frozen vegetables. These staples make it easy to create quick, healthy meals.

How can I maintain variety in my meals and avoid getting bored?

Rotate ingredients and explore new recipes regularly. Try different cuisines, experiment with spice combinations, or swap out your usual proteins and vegetables for seasonal ones. Batch cooking with different variations also helps keep meals exciting throughout the week.

References and Helpful Links

Maher, D. (2025, April 11). Consider salt sensitivity in women's midlife blood pressure management. Medscape.
https://www.medscape.com/viewarticle/consider-salt-sensitivity-womens-midlife-blood-pressure-2025a10008p

Aging may worsen the effects of a high-salt diet. (2016, February 16). ScienceDaily.
https://www.sciencedaily.com/releases/2016/02/160209122608.htm

Clinic, C. (2025, April 23). How to add flavor to your food without salt. Cleveland Clinic.
https://health.clevelandclinic.org/know-salt-hiding-food#:~:text=It%20does%20help%20to%20avoid,Frozen%20meals.

Rd, J. K. M. (2025, April 28). Your guide to the low sodium diet. Healthline. https://www.healthline.com/nutrition/low-sodium-diet

Low-sodium recipes - Mayo Clinic. (n.d.).
https://www.mayoclinic.org/healthy-lifestyle/recipes/low-sodium-recipes/rcs-20077197

Rd, J. K. (2024, August 6). The best 25 High-Protein, Low-Sodium snacks for your health. Health.
https://www.health.com/high-protein-low-sodium-snacks-8673928

Glander, A. (2024, September 18). 43 Low-Sodium recipes that are kind to your heart. Taste of Home. https://www.tasteofhome.com/collection/low-sodium-recipes/

7-Day Low-Sodium Meal Plan: Easy, healthy, and delicious. (n.d.). https://www.cookunity.com/blog/low-sodium-diet-meal-plan?srsltid=AfmBOopT12JLlSSnhNVcVnif_vaQMCW8MHN66hHVodh1X2Rr750JkorG